NEEM

MARIAN KIM

ISBN: 1508667101

ISBN-13: 978-1508667100

CONTENTS

1

PROPERTIES

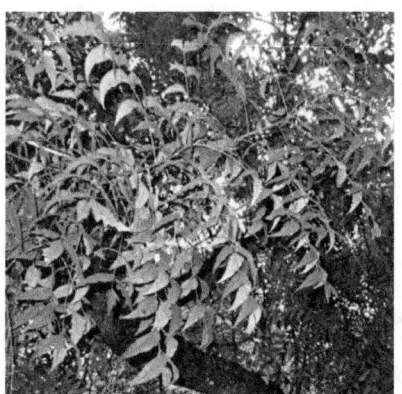

Scientific name: Azadirachta indica

Other names: Arishta, bead tree, holy tree, Indian lilac, pride of China, mwarobaini

Properties

Anti-inflammatory properties

Antiseptic (antibacterial, antiviral, antifungal) properties

Antipyretic (fever reducing) properties

Analgesic (pain relieving) properties

Astringent properties

Immunostimulant (immune boosting) properties

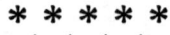

2

USES

Medically Proven Uses

Insect repellent

Neem oil has been shown in a study to be more effective than DEET as an insect repellent. It is used to repel mosquitos.

***

Other Uses

Lice treatment

Neem is used to treat head lice. 5 ml of neem oil can be mixed with 5 ml of a carrier oil like olive oil to make a scalp massage oil. This oil should be massaged onto the scalp and hair and left for at least 1 hour before being shampooed. This treatment should be repeated weekly for at least 3 weeks.

Dandruff treatment

Neem is used to treat dandruff. Neem oil can be added to shampoo to help get rid of dandruff.

Cuts, wounds and skin ulcer treatment

Neem leaves and fruit are used to treat ulcers on the skin as well as wounds.

Wart treatment

Neem oil is used to treat warts. 1 drop of the neat neem oil can be applied on the wart once per day for at least 2 weeks.

Acne treatment

Neem can be used both topically (applied on the skin) or orally (taken by mouth) to treat acne naturally. Neem oil is extracted from crushed seeds of the neem tree. It has anti-inflammatory properties which are useful for managing the inflammation associated with acne. It also soothes inflamed skin without irritating it. This oil can be applied on the skin or used to make soaps and moisturizers for natural acne treatment. Neem oil also has skin antiseptic (antibacterial) properties which are useful for treating acne. It also has astringent properties. Poultices made from neem leaves are also used to treat acne.

Athlete's foot treatment

Neem oil has antifungal properties and it is used to treat athlete's foot. 3 teaspoons of neem oil can be added to a bowl of warm water to soak the feet and treat athlete's foot. Neem oil can also be diluted with a carrier oil and used to treat athlete's foot.

Ringworm treatment

Neem has antifungal properties and it is used to treat ringworms. Neem oil can also be diluted with a carrier oil and used to treat ringworms.

Eczema and psoriasis treatment

Neem oil which has anti-inflammatory properties are useful for managing the inflammation associated with eczema and psoriasis. It also soothes inflamed skin without irritating it. Neem oil can also be used to make soaps and moisturizers for natural eczema and psoriasis treatment.

Cold sores treatment

Neem has antiviral properties and it is used to treat cold sores.

Diabetes treatment

Neem leaves, fruits and twigs are used to treat diabetes.

High blood pressure treatment

Neem is used to treat high blood pressure.

Leprosy treatment

Neem leaves, fruit, seed and seed oil are used to treat leprosy.

Eye disorders treatment

Neem leaf is used to treat eye disorders. Neem fruit is also used to treat eye disorders.

Intestinal worms treatment

Neem leaves, flowers, fruits, twigs, seeds and seed oil are used to treat intestinal worms.

Upset stomach treatment

Neem leaf is used to treat upset stomachs.

Anorexia treatment

Neem leaf is used to treat anorexia or loss of appetite.

Fever treatment

Neem leaf is used to treat fever. Neem bark is also used for fever.

Gingivitis treatment

Neem leaf extract is used to treat gingivitis which is a gum disease.

Contraceptive

Neem leaf and seed oil is used as a contraceptive. Neem creams made with at least 25% neem oil are also used as contraceptives.

Malaria treatment

Neem bark is used to treat malaria.

Stomach ulcers treatment

Neem bark extract is used to treat stomach and intestinal ulcers. Studies show that it helps them heal.

Hemorrhoid treatment

Neem fruits and twigs are used to treat hemorrhoids.

Urinary tract disorder treatment

Neem fruits and twigs are used to treat urinary tract disorders.

Coughs and asthma treatment

Neem twigs are used to treat coughs and asthma. Neem flowers and fruit are also used for controlling phlegm.

Sensitive skin soother

Neem is used to soothe sensitive skin

Hair loss treatment

Neem is used to manage thinning hair and hair loss disorder treatment. Neem oil is also used to manage damaged hair.

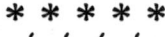

3

SAFETY PRECAUTIONS

1. Neem oil should not be taken by mouth.

2. Persons who are allergic to aspirin should not take neem.

3. Children should not use neem. Side effects associated with children using neem oil include diarrhea, vomiting, convulsions, drowsiness, coma and death.

4. Pregnant women should not use herbal remedies with neem oil and neem bark since they can cause miscarriages.

5. Persons trying to conceive should not use/avoid neem since it can damage sperms and cause miscarriages.

6. Persons with autoimmune diseases like systemic lupus erythematosus (SLE or lupus), multiple sclerosis (MS) and rheumatoid arthritis should not use/avoid neem since it can worsen them.

7. Persons who have had organ transplants should not use neem since it might reduce the effectiveness of the medications used to prevent organ rejection.

8. Persons with diabetes should not use neem since it can lower blood glucose levels.

9. Persons scheduled to have surgery should not use/avoid neem since it can lower blood glucose levels during and after the surgery.

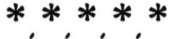

4

DRUG INTERACTIONS

1. Persons using lithium should not use /avoid neem.

2. Persons using diabetes medications should not use /avoid neem since it can also lower blood glucose levels.

3. Persons using immunosuppressants (medications which suppress the immune system) should not use /avoid neem since it can decrease their effectivneness. Examples of such medications include azathioprine (Imuran), cyclosporine (Neoral), prednisone (Deltasone) and tacrolimus.

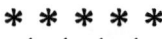

5

HERBAL RECIPES

Neem Tea

Equipment

Tea pot or kettle

***

Ingredients

1 teaspoon of finely crushed or minced neem leaves or 4-5 fresh neem leaves

1 cup of boiling water

Honey to taste (optional)

***

Instructions

1. Put the neem leaves in a tea pot or kettle, add the boiling water and let it steep while covered for 5 -15 minutes.

2. Strain the leaves and add honey (if using) to suit your taste before drinking.

***

Tips

1. Neem tea can be used as a face wash for acne prone skin.

*****

Neem Tincture

Equipment

Glass jar with tight fitting lid

Dark tincture bottles

Cheesecloth

***

Ingredients

7 oz (200 gm) of dried neem leaves or 14 oz (400 gm) of fresh neem leaves

30 oz (1 liter) of 80-100 proof vodka

***

Instructions

1. Fill 1/3 of the glass jar with the neem.

2. Add the vodka to completely fill the jar to the top.

3. Seal the jar and label it with the date of preparation and name of botanical (neem) used.

4. Store the glass jar in a dark place for 6 weeks ensuring that you shake them weekly.

5. After 6 weeks strain out the neem with a cheesecloth and pour the tincture into dark tincture bottles.

6. Label the tincture bottles and tore them away from light and heat.

*****

Neem Poultice

Equipment

Cheesecloth or old cotton sheet strips

***

Ingredients

1 tablespoon mashed, fresh neem leaves or powdered, dry neem leaves

Boiling water

***

Instructions

1. Add enough boiling water to the neem leaves to wet it and make a thick paste.

2. Spoon the neem leaves paste onto the cheesecloth (or bed sheet strips) to make the poultice.

3. To use, apply the poultice to the affected area and cover with another piece of hot, wet cloth. Replace the hot, wet cloth when it cools with another hot one to keep the poultice hot.

***

Tips

1. Add 1 teaspoon of turmeric to make and acne treatment poultice.

*****

Neem Massage Oil

Equipment

Dark glass or plastic bottle

***

Ingredients

50 ml carrier oil like organic olive, sweet almond oil or sunflower oil

5 ml neem oil

10 drops essential oils like lavender (optional natural fragrance)

***

Instructions

1. Mix the neem oil, carrier oil and essential oil in the bottle.

***

Tips

1. Neem massage oil can be used as an insect repellent. It can also be used to treat eczema, psoriasis, cold sores, fungal infections like athlete's foot and ringworms. Neem massage oil can also be applied to minor cuts or wounds.

*****

Neem Infused Oil

Equipment

Double boiler

Large glass bowl

Sieve and cheesecloth

Sterilized dark jars

***

Ingredients

16 fl oz. (500 ml) vegetable oil like organic olive, sweet almond oil or sunflower oil

8 oz. (250 grams) slightly crushed, dry neem leaves or 16 oz. (500 grams) slightly bruised fresh neem leaves

***

Instructions

1. Place the neem leaves and oil in the glass bowl ensuring that the oil covers the neem. Simmer them in a double boiler for 1 hour at around 120 degrees Fahrenheit (49 degrees Celsius). Do not let the mixture boil. You can repeat this step several times after letting the oils cool to create more concentrated herb infused oils.

2. Strain the mixture with a sieve and cheesecloth into a dark jar as you squeeze out as much oil as you can from the cheesecloth.

3. Label your jars and store your neem infused oils in a cool dark place or in the refrigerator and use them within 3 months.

*****

Neem Salve

Equipment

Double boiler

Large glass bowl

Sterilized dark jars or tins

***

Ingredients

8 oz. (250 ml or 1 cup) neem infused vegetable oil (see previous recipe)

1 oz. (30 grams) beeswax

10 drops essential oils like tea tree or lavender essential oil (optional natural fragrance)

***

Instructions

1. Place the beeswax and neem infused oil in the glass bowl and melt them in a double boiler.

2. Once melted remove from the heat source, allow to cool and add the essential oils (if using).

3. Pour the melted oils into the storage jars or tins and allow to cool completely.

4. Store the salves in a cool dark place.

***

Tips

1. Neem salve can also be made by melting ½ oz. (15 grams) of beeswax with 2 oz. (60 ml) of olive oil and 2 oz (60 ml) of neem oil in a

double boiler. The mixture is removed from the heat source once the beeswax melts and poured into storage tins.

###

ABOUT THE AUTHOR

Marian Kim is an experienced alternative medicine practitioner.

OTHER BOOKS BY THE AUTHOR

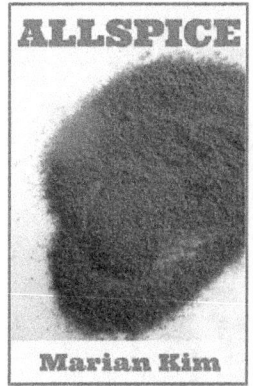

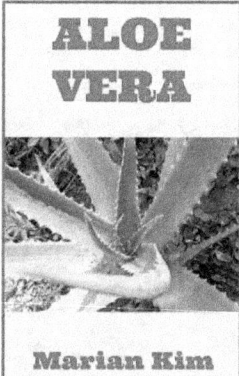

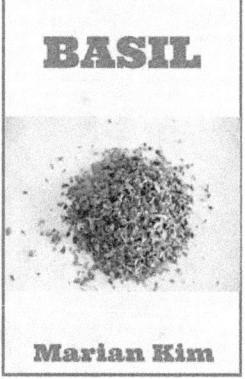

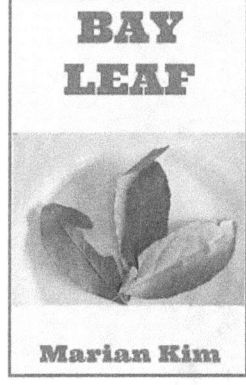

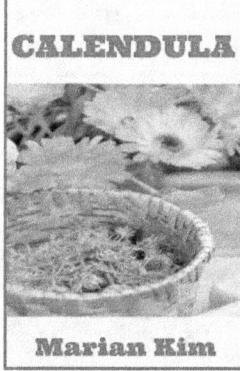

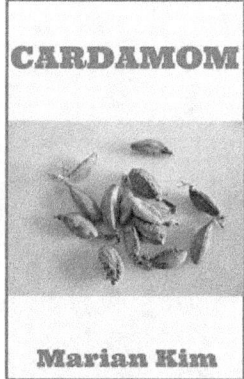

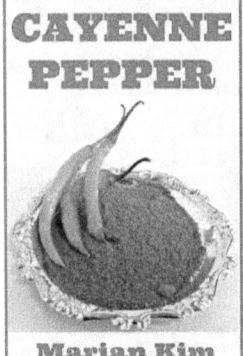
CAYENNE PEPPER
Marian Kim

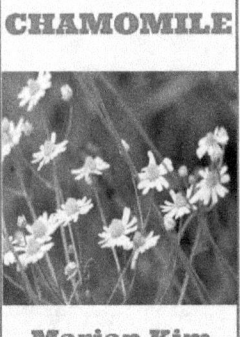
CHAMOMILE
Marian Kim

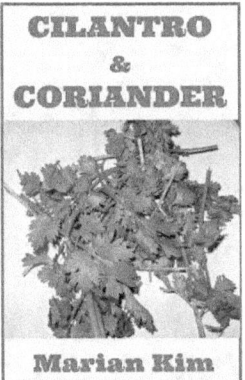
CILANTRO & CORIANDER
Marian Kim

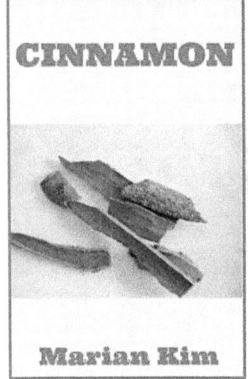
CINNAMON
Marian Kim

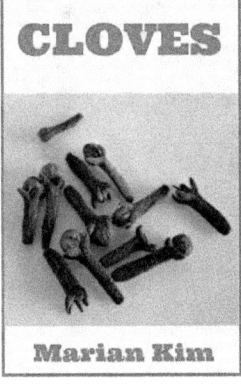
CLOVES
Marian Kim

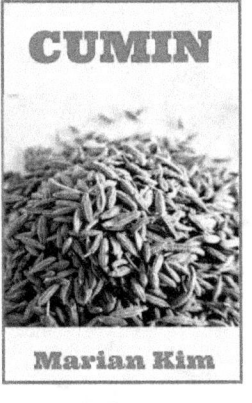
CUMIN
Marian Kim

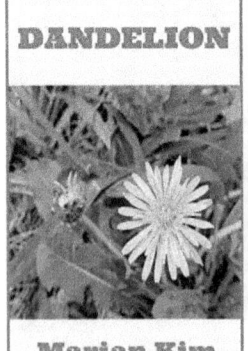
DANDELION
Marian Kim

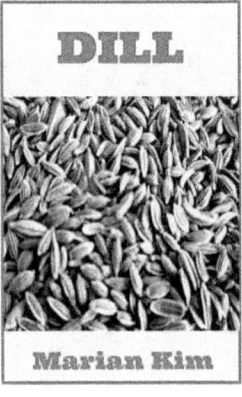
DILL
Marian Kim

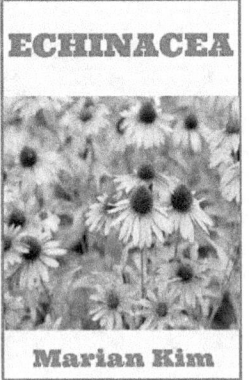
ECHINACEA
Marian Kim

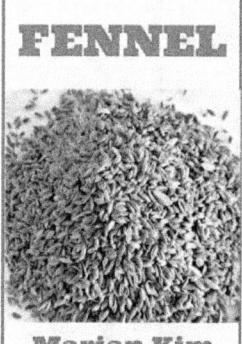
FENNEL

Marian Kim

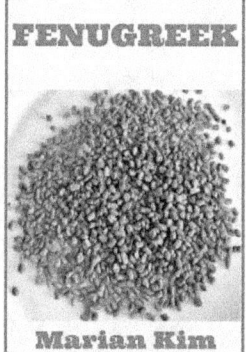
FENUGREEK

Marian Kim

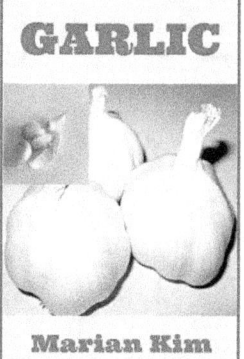
GARLIC

Marian Kim

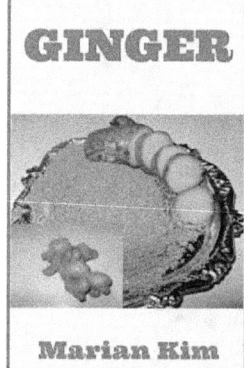
GINGER

Marian Kim

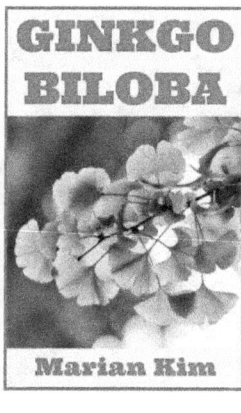
GINKGO BILOBA

Marian Kim

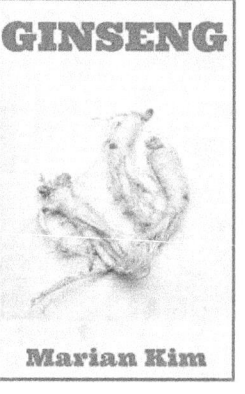
GINSENG

Marian Kim

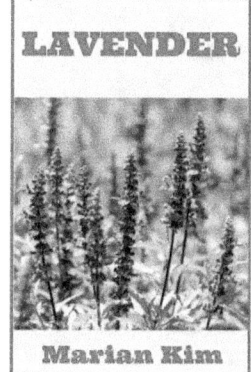
LAVENDER

Marian Kim

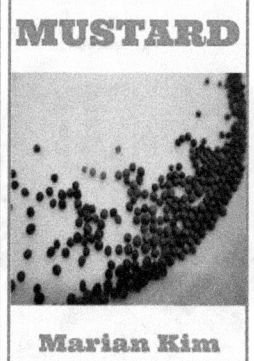
MUSTARD

Marian Kim

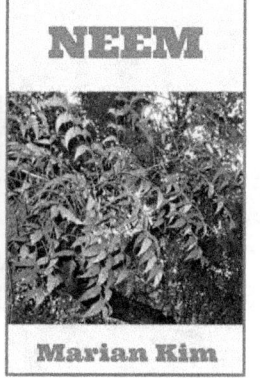
NEEM

Marian Kim

NUTMEG & MACE

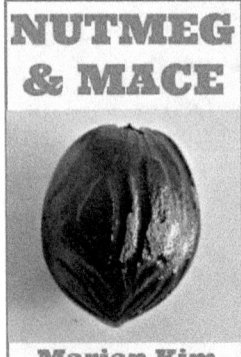

Marian Kim

OREGANO

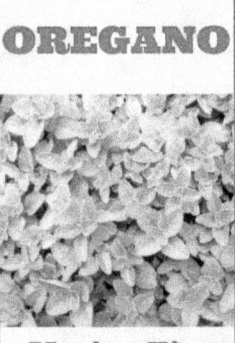

Marian Kim

PAPRIKA

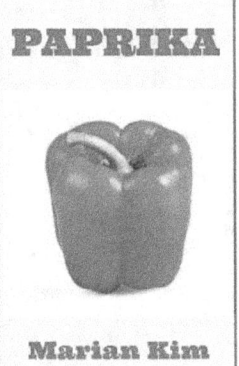

Marian Kim

PARSLEY

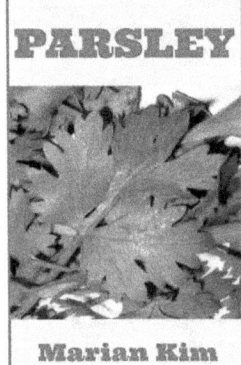

Marian Kim

BLACK & WHITE PEPPER

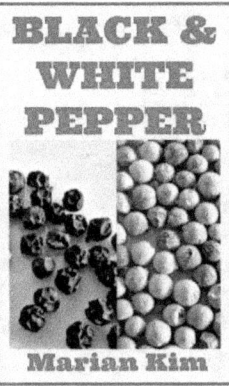

Marian Kim

PEPPERMINT

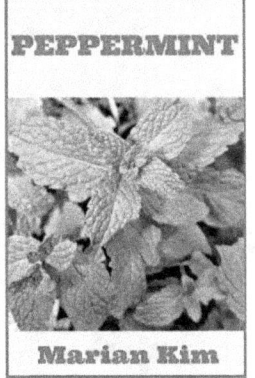

Marian Kim

ROSE HIPS

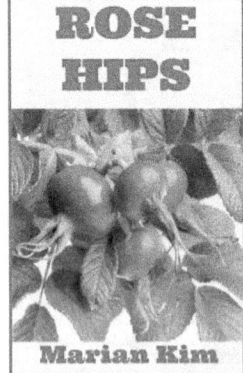

Marian Kim

ROSE PETALS

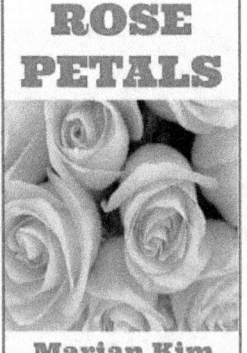

Marian Kim

ROSEMARY

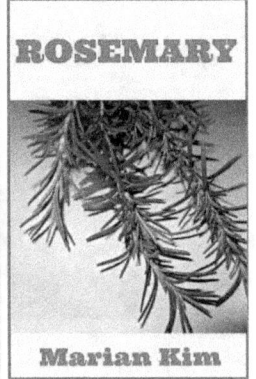

Marian Kim

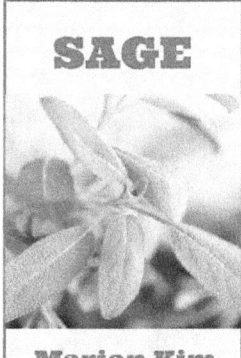
SAGE
Marian Kim

ST. JOHN'S WORT
Marian Kim

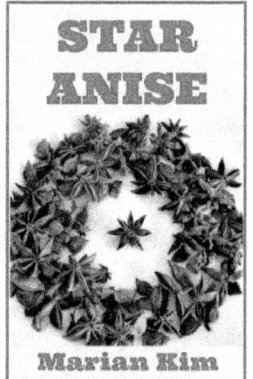
STAR ANISE
Marian Kim

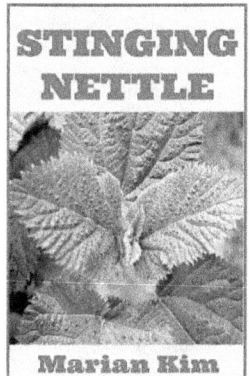
STINGING NETTLE
Marian Kim

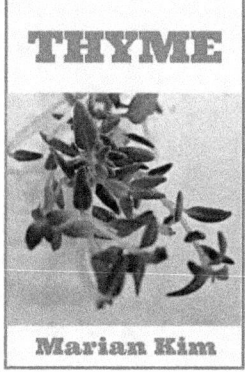
THYME
Marian Kim

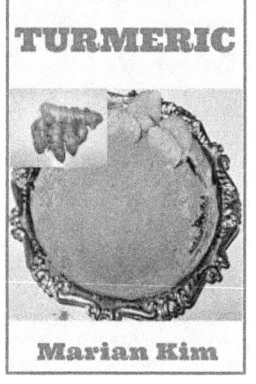
TURMERIC
Marian Kim

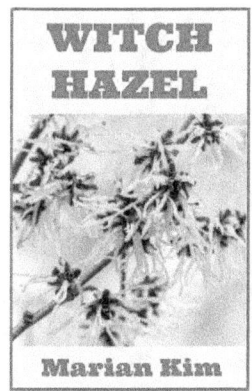
WITCH HAZEL
Marian Kim

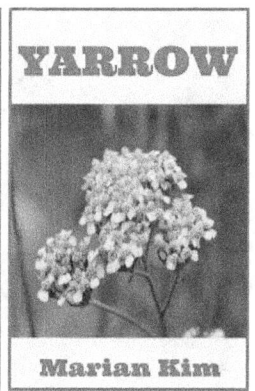
YARROW
Marian Kim

*****

www.ingramcontent.com/pod-product-compliance
Lightning Source LLC
Chambersburg PA
CBHW071345310526
45790CB00018B/1369

* 9 7 8 1 5 0 8 6 6 7 1 0 0 *